Living the best life with Fibromyalgia

Alisha Nurse M.A

Table of Contents

For Sue Jacobs,
& to my fellow fibromyalgia friends
who are fighting for their lives.

Note to the Reader

This book does not provide medical advice. The suggestions shared in this work reflect what's worked for the author. Please consult with your doctor before starting any new treatments.

Introduction

"The good life is one inspired by love and guided by knowledge"
— Bertrand Russell

In 2010, I was 25 when a rheumatologist diagnosed me with fibromyalgia (fms)[1].

A wave of intense emotion washed over me. Not because I was distraught, it was all down to overwhelming relief. You see, since my childhood I had been subject to endless doctor visits, blood tests and examinations to determine the cause of pain, debilitating exhaustion, lack of sleep and other symptoms that I suffered. It was all to no avail. Scraping through life without an explanation and treatment proved difficult. In childhood I was often absent from school and in adulthood, I had no reason for employers when I was too unwell to work. My social life was non-existent.

Years after my diagnosis, I became far worse before I got any better. It's been a long road to reaching this point and after receiving much positive feedback from my blog about living with fibromyalgia, I decided to write this handbook

---

1   Abbreviated form of fibromyalgia.

highlighting some of the things that have worked for me in my fight against this chronic, misunderstood condition.

Fibro-who?

When I first heard the word, I never believed that I would learn to say it with such ease. Try saying it slowly: fi-bro-my-al-gia.

Fibromyalgia. There.

Fibromyalgia is a neurological condition characterised by "widespread musculoskeletal pain accompanied by fatigue, sleep, memory and mood issues."[2] Other symptoms include chronic headaches, depression and anxiety, irritable bowel syndrome, Multiple Chemical Sensitivity Syndrome (sensitivities to noise, bright lights, chemicals, medications or foods), cognitive difficulties (also called fibro fog), allodynia (feeling pain from things that shouldn't be painful, like tickles or the feel of clothes against one's skin) and hyperalgesia (extreme sensitivity to pain).

No one knows for certain what causes fibromyalgia, but leading research efforts into this condition suggest that the most common cause is positional cervical cord compression[3], found in 71 percent of fms patients.

---

2   Mayo Clinic mayoclinic.org/diseases-conditions/fibromyalgia/basics/definition/con-20019243

3   fmpartnership.org/articles/PC3_Holman.pdf

In the lead up to my diagnosis, one doctor emphatically told me that I "might have fibromyalgia, but be thankful you're not dying of cancer."

It was particularly painful to hear these words. While doctors say fibromyalgia is not life threatening, in many ways it is. Fibromyalgia might not directly cause death but it leaves so many patients mere shadows of their former selves, robbing their lives of all things good and fulfilling.

I was grateful that I didn't have a terminal condition. However, many days I was bed bound, immobilised by overwhelming exhaustion and requiring help to lift myself up. Just the act of getting out of bed knocked the wind out of me, and simple tasks like combing my hair or having a shower left me out of breath, needing a break.

I was at university doing my Masters Degree at the time and it was a common thing to find me slumped on desks, fast asleep as I suffered a kind of sleep paralysis, unable to wake myself until my body said it was ready.

"Is Alisha alright?" I would hear my classmates asking but I couldn't pull myself out of the deep slumber to answer.

I was desperate for answers. I was 25 and I felt like my life had ended before it began.

Not surprisingly, research conducted by Dr Lene Dreyer, a rheumatologist at Copenhagen University Hospital found that a "significant" number of fibromyalgia patients tend to die from suicide, which she linked to depression.

I joined support groups for people living with fibromyalgia and I learned about the problems patients were having at work, with family and in their romantic relationships due to their diagnosis. I heard of marriages breaking down, cheating spouses and families calling their loved ones lazy or liars. It wasn't unfamiliar to me. I too had been called lazy, criticised for my constant drowsiness and accused of "not making an effort" in relationships.

Not too long after my first diagnosis, I saw a second rheumatologist at a Fibromyalgia Clinic in London, and he confirmed my diagnosis. He took the time to explain the condition, provide me with literature, and a long list of suggestions, which he asked my general practitioner to implement. These included referrals for physiotherapy and psychotherapy (to treat depression). That was when I started to get a clearer understanding of this condition which affects 1 in 25 people in the UK, according to Arthritis Research UK. From there it was a rough road but it's only gotten better, with a few bumpy patches in between. I still suffer terribly when my symptoms flare but this typically happens during stressful periods, and when the seasons are changing.

It is imperative that I point out the suggestions mentioned in this book are not medical advice. I am not a medical professional. I am simply a fibromyalgia patient who is sharing what has worked for me over the years.

It is a journey which I am still on, and I have far to go. However I can see the major progress I've made and if I can do it, then so can you. It is my hope that my story will give you strength to walk on, with courage and hope.

Challenges

"The gem cannot be polished without friction, nor man perfected without trials" – Chinese proverb

Living with fibromyalgia presents many challenges. The range of symptoms is so varied, and many of these seem to need individual treatments for their management. This means more medication which many patients find difficult to manage with fibro fog, and without help.

Personally I have been harping on to the general practitioner about my debilitating exhaustion, literally begging for a suggestion of medication or supplement that will help. Each of us battles our demon symptom, the one symptom that is king above all else. For me, that's the chronic exhaustion. But my GP says there is nothing she can recommend except for exercise.

Fibromyalgia creates vicious cycles in patients. My GP believes I will feel better and improve my exhaustion levels if I can get some exercise. The problem is that I am often too fatigued to do the simplest of tasks, so the idea of exercise is terrifying. At the gym I have only been able to manage 15 minutes by completely pushing myself, and I felt like I was on the brink of collapse. So I am not motivated to go to the gym but I try to get some stretches and basic steps done at home. Ideally I'd opt for swimming but I can't swim (yet). Exercise would also help my issue of gaining weight (probably from medication). The more weight I gain, the more tired I feel. It becomes harder to physically move and my mood goes lower. As a result, I comfort eat, I gain more weight and exercise becomes even harder.

Eating healthy might appear difficult when a lot of us are only managing to meet the very minimum requirements to survive. Unless one lives with family members to help prepare meals, I imagine breakfast, lunch and dinner might mean pre-packaged or unhealthy fast foods.

The issues of chronic pain and debilitating exhaustion mean that many fibromyalgia patients are forced to quit their jobs, unable to work or attend school. This is another kind of cycle that perpetuates symptoms. At times when I'm really unwell and stuck in bed I find that my knees and muscles get weaker, and it becomes harder to get up and about. I end up feeling wearier. Physical movement becomes more difficult but without it, the stiffer and weaker my muscles get.

Many of us get easily stressed, and that's understandable. When one is in pain, so exhausted, and noises seem right next to one's ears (due to increased sensitivity) it's hard not to get irritable. Anything else just piles on the stress.

Controversies surrounding the legitimacy and cause of fibromyalgia result in some doctors being reluctant to treat patients. I still hear stories within support groups from patients who say their doctors don't believe them. It is a humiliating experience yes, but equally, a limiting action which prevents patients from getting the care and treatment that they need.

On the issue of doubters, many patients also find themselves facing up to sceptical family members or partners. I've heard fibromyalgia patients say their children, in-laws, spouses and even friends accuse them of faking their symptoms, or being lazy. One girl recently told my support group that her neighbour had reported her to a hotline for people with information on someone committing benefit fraud, or misusing support from social services. The idea was that the girl couldn't be unfit for work because she looked well on the outside. The breakdown of relationships due to a diagnosis is just an unnecessary stress that no patient needs.

Another challenge I've faced that other fms patients I know have experienced is the situation where fibromyalgia impacts on romantic relationships. Some years ago when I decided to try out dating, I found myself in a conundrum. I didn't know when the right time was to tell the other party about fms. I sometimes told myself 'I'll do it next time I see him' but eventually, and inevitably, I had to spit it out. It was usually because I had cancelled a meeting due to feeling unwell, or I was so exhausted and in pain on a date that I couldn't hide it. Some took it well but others didn't. After my dating experience I decided that even though I didn't like it, fibromyalgia was a part of my life and any potential partner should know. I now encourage others to do the same because I feel it's best for both parties. You can find out whether the person is ok with it from the onset to avoid later hurt. Also, by being upfront about it, you allow yourself the freedom to just be you, unmasked. You don't have to hide how you're feeling or pretend.

Other patients I know have mentioned their marriages with unsupportive spouses. Now, I'm no marriage counsellor but I think we have a duty to ourselves to address relationship issues when they start impacting on our health. If after the conversations no change is happening, walk on. It's not easy and I imagine it is harder when one is married and children are involved. I've had to move on from some relationships, and it wasn't easy when emotions threatened to take me over, but those were some of the best decisions I made. I learnt that I don't benefit from unsupportive people in my life, and it helped me to appreciate the people who are supportive. Just like one might do an internal cleanse, a social cleanse is imperative. It is ridding your life of all the unnecessary weeds.

Living with an invisible illness is a challenge in itself. There is no physical marker or sign of disability, so people living with fibromyalgia often encounter critics who question whether or not we are unwell. A common problem experienced by my friends is the scenario where members of the public challenge patients who are parked in disabled bays (even with a disabled badge!). In the past I have felt that I almost had to prove that I was unwell to disbelieving people close to me. No one who is unwell should ever feel compelled to prove their condition to another.

I know this collection of challenges is daunting, and this is by no means an extensive list. It is easy to want to give up on life, but I really need you to consider an idea that I will expound on later. Sometimes it is the very things that we consider impediments in our lives that end up pushing us forward.

Diet

"A healthy outside starts from the inside" – Robert Urich

Soon after my second diagnosis, one of the first things I did was re-evaluate my diet. From the age of 10 I had become pesco-vegetarian. I had grown up eating healthily with only fresh foods from my grampie's garden, but in my post university years I had fallen into the trap of loving processed, pre-packaged foods and fast foods. I considered my healthy nintey-something year old grandparents, and thought it was worth readopting my former diet.

It was trying at first but I began by cutting out processed and fast foods. By processed foods I mean things like bread, pasta, canned vegetables, canned meats, frozen foods (I ate a lot of frozen pizzas), cereals, savoury snacks, and soft drinks. Then I cut out the fast foods (by this I mean burgers, chips, milkshakes, kebabs...). I'd learnt that processed and fast foods don't necessarily have to be unhealthy but most times these foods contain higher amounts of sugar, salt and calories ultimately. These foods didn't seem like the healthiest options if I was going to fix my diet and manage a healthy weight. While making these cuts I increased the amount of fresh fruit, vegetables and fish I ate, finding a cheap source from vendors at the market. I increased my intake of filtered water, and I cut out the snacks – ice cream, cakes, biscuits, sweets, nachos... Ever so often when I break my bread rule and indulge in it, I see a flare in symptoms related to irritable bowel syndrome (IBS).

If like me you also struggle with intense tummy pains due to IBS, another symptom associated with fibromyalgia, it may be worth cutting out or lessening your intake of gluten and dairy products. Whole milk makes me bloat terribly so I only use soy milk. Admittedly I am a great lover of cheese which I refuse to give up so I try to have that in moderation.

In recent times I have taken up the ketogenic diet[4], which consists of eating mostly natural fats (greek yogurts, fish, cheeses, eggs), moderate protein and low carbohydrates (less than 20 grams a day). There are lots of resources online on this and I follow a simple guide which sees me thinking like a caveman. If it's pre-packaged, or has been refined in some way then it's probably not natural so it doesn't fit into my diet plan. I avoid the 0% fat products as these tend to have higher sugar content. Again, please remember that I am not a doctor so if you are considering this diet, make sure and check in with your doctor first. It takes discipline and every now and again I fall back into bad habits, but within two

---

4   ketogenic-diet-resource.com

weeks I started seeing benefits, which included weight loss, improved digestion and reduced IBS symptoms.

Say no to...

I've also been learning the importance of cooking with healthy oils like coconut and olive oils. I always bought the cheaper cooking oils like sunflower and vegetable oils, before I learnt of their reputation for triggering inflammation in the body. This is due to the presence of Omega 6 Fatty Acids (not to be confused with Omega 3 Fatty Acids which are good for us). While our bodies need Omega 6 fatty acids, excessive amounts are harmful to us, triggering the production of inflammatory chemicals. These are found in peanut oil, vegetable, corn, soy, sunflower and grapeseed oils, as well as in many salad dressings and mayonnaise.

I often think that if I focus too hard on what I'm eating, there'd be nothing left to eat! However I believe that at least having an awareness of what's good and what's not, can help us to limit the foods that cause harm to our bodies. Trans fats are considered the worst kind of fat out there.[5] They trigger an inflammatory effect in the body. In case you don't know, Trans fats are formed during a process that adds hydrogen to vegetable oil. This oil is less likely to go off, and

5   mayoclinic.org/diseases-conditions/high-blood-cholesterol/in-depth/trans-fat/art-20046114

foods with it tend have a longer shelf life (that's one hint in what to avoid). These fats are everywhere, in potato crisps, biscuits, cakes, frozen pizza crusts, margarine, and foods that are deep fried like chips and doughnuts. It is worth doing some reading online to see the comprehensive list of foods with Trans fats. I've also reduced my intake of Saturated fat. These raise our cholesterol levels and are present in whole milk, ice creams, cakes, sausages, cheeses and butter. Women are meant to have no more than 20 grams a days, while men are allowed 30 grams. The NHS has a useful guide[6] on eating less Saturated fat.

One of the hardest things I've had to do was reduce the amount of sugar I consume. Sugar is another culprit known to trigger the release of inflammatory messengers in our bodies. I didn't always know this and when I endeavoured to cut back, it was for entirely different reasons. I grew up in a house where tea was cherished. I would see my relatives pouring condensed milk freely into our pot of breakfast tea every morning, and I grew up with a love of all things sweet. In my later years I couldn't enjoy a cup of tea without at least three teaspoons of sugar, but when my weight gain started spiralling out of control, I knew that I needed to put a handle on it. It was hard, and sometimes I cheated by adding a little extra sugar when no one was looking. Silly I know, but I soon realised that I was only cheating myself! I

6   nhs.uk/Livewell/Goodfood/Pages/Eat-less-saturated-fat.aspx

eventually went down to two teaspoons of sugar, then down to one. If I'm feeling particularly weak the most I allow myself is one and a half spoons of sugar in my tea. I've gotten used to the taste now, and that's really helped me to manage with cutting down sugar in other foods. It's hard to avoid sugar when it's in everything we purchase. That's one of the reasons why I try my best to limit my intake of packaged foods, cereals and deserts, even the ones that claim to be healthy.

Numerous other foods are known to cause inflammation in the body. Many of them mentioned previously at the beginning of this chapter. These include mono-sodium glutamate (MSG), refined carbohydrates like white flour and potatoes, gluten, Aspartame, excessive alcohol and whole milk.

Throughout this book, you will find me naming the same culprits and winners. They are worth remembering so you can start changing your diet. The thing is we can't act on what we don't know, so it's crucial to familiarise ourselves with the good, the bad and the ugly foods.

Below I have outlined some key foods that I make an effort to include in my diet to manage fibromyalgia.

Full Fat Greek Yogurts & Peppermint

I was never a fan of yogurts but I started trying to have a small portion at least once a day or every other day to help with irritable bowel syndrome. Many fibromyalgia patients I've spoken to experience either severe constipation or diarrhoea. For me it's always been the former and I tried everything including prescriptions from my GP. It can be quite distressing but I found full fat Greek yogurt to be very effective. Yogurts with probiotics work to manage a healthy gut via certain bacterial strains (*B. infantis* and *L. Acidophilus).* They reduce pain, inflammation and bloating. In addition to this, when I can, I take an Acidophilus supplement, which I purchase from a local health shop. I don't really like peppermint tea but this is another helpful food in battling IBS. I take one peppermint capsule three times a day. The menthol in peppermint is also said to be useful in preventing muscle spasms, which a lot of us experience.

Ginger

Known as a natural painkiller and anti-inflammatory food, ginger has always been recommended by my grandmother for pain. In particular she would insist that I drink a strong cup of ginger tea (for this recipe and others see the next section). I usually drink at least one cup a couple times a week but I use it as often as needed. Apart from being an awesome pain reliever, this root spice has also provided me with effective relief from irritable bowel syndrome and nausea. It's also reputed to be useful in treating migraines which is a common symptom of fibromyalgia. It's been so helpful that I always keep fresh ginger at home, and some crystallised ginger in my handbag for bloating/gas emergencies or when I feel nauseous when I'm out. Ginger is also said to relieve dizziness which I also grapple with. I use lots of ginger in my home cooking. It's particularly great in stir fries and curries.

Turmeric

Known for its anti-inflammatory properties, turmeric is a natural pain reliever. It is also useful for digestion problems. You're probably familiar with it for its use in curries, but when I was growing up it was commonly used by women in my family as a natural internal cleanser. My relatives would buy the fresh root in the market, grate it and bring to boil. They would then strain and sweeten it (milk is optional) to enjoy a tasty cup of tea. I still do this particularly when I have a cold or I'm achy. It works wonders thanks to the substance in turmeric called curcumin. I purchase fresh turmeric online, grate it and freeze it, so it's there whenever I need it. Sometimes I drop a tablespoon of it in my peanut butter smoothie with soy milk. If like me you also live with acid reflux disease then it's important to have this in moderation, or at least know when you've had enough.

Vitamin D/calcium

Vitamin D strengthens our muscles, teeth and bones. It's needed for the absorption and utilisation of calcium in our bodies. Following hospitalisation, I was found to have low vitamin D levels. My GP placed me on a supplement. I was surprised to learn that many other fms patients in my online support group also suffered this deficiency. Low levels of vitamin D are associated with high levels of chronic pain. I still take a supplement but I also try to ensure I eat vitamin D rich foods like oily fish and eggs.

Magnesium

Though the evidence is mixed, some studies have suggested that magnesium supplements might be helpful in managing fibromyalgia and pain levels. Magnesium supplements form part of my health regime, and as with everything else mentioned, I try to ensure a decent intake of foods rich in this mineral. Magnesium is found in a number of foods like green leafy vegetables (my favourite is pak choi), nuts, wholegrain breads, fish, meat and dairy foods. Just think fibre. If it's rich in fibre, it's likely loaded with magnesium.

Cinnamon

Studies have found that this antioxidant-rich spice reduces inflammation and improves brain function. I absolutely love cinnamon, and I use it liberally in my curries, sometimes adding it to my pot of boiling ginger tea. You can add this versatile spice to your diet in many ways. Sprinkle a dash of cinnamon on your morning coffee or tea, oatmeal porridge or full fat greek yogurt. Cinnamon has been found to have benefits in improving diabetes and Parkinson's disease. This old spice, rich in fibre, alleviates symptoms associated with irritable bowel syndrome. Cinnamon is a must- have spice in our diets for managing fibro fog, muscle pains and IBS.

Fish & Omega 3 fatty acids

I had long been advised by a rheumatologist at the Fibromyalgia Clinic that eating foods rich in omega 3 fatty acids would be effective in managing fibromyalgia, due to their anti-inflammatory effects. I take a supplement but I also try to eat a lot of oily fish like mackerel and salmon. All fish have omega 3 oils but salmon, herrings and anchovies are loaded with them. Research has shown that omega 3 oils are beneficial to increasing blood flow and reducing inflammation. They're also useful for elevating the mood, and managing cardiovascular health. Doctors recommend eating fish at least twice a week.

Antioxidant foods

Think blueberries, cherries, tomatoes, spinach, sweet peppers and squash, all the colourful fruits and vegetables. I usually eat a bowl of blueberries or seasonal fruit in the morning, and ensure that antioxidant rich foods are incorporated into my cooking. Antioxidant rich foods are known to be helpful the treatment in many conditions. While research has not specifically indicated that they are beneficial for the treatment of fibromyalgia, studies have shown that they are beneficial to our health in the long term. Antioxidants are known for cleaning up free radicals in the body, associated with triggering numerous degenerative diseases.

Recipes

"To keep the body in good health is a duty, otherwise we shall not be able to keep our mind strong and clear" – Buddha

Following on from the last section, I've compiled some recipes for dishes that include some of the key foods we need to manage fibromyalgia. I've been eating some of these meals since childhood. I hope you enjoy!

Ginger tea

Ingredients

Finger sized piece of ginger
3 cups of water
A few drops of lemon or lime

Method

Grate ginger with the skin on and toss in a pot with water.

Bring to boil and simmer for at least 15 minutes. If the tea is too strong you can add more water but I always feel the stronger it is the more effective!

Strain and sweeten with honey or a little sugar. Add a few drops of lemon or lime if you like

Sip while hot. It's a herbal remedy that works wonders for achy muscles, joints and the flu!

Reuse the ginger to make more tea.

Turmeric tea

Ingredients

A handful of grated turmeric root
3 cups water
Milk/sugar to taste

Method

Toss grated turmeric in pot with water and bring to boil for at least 15-20 minutes.

Strain and sweeten, adding a splash of soy milk. I cheat and add a few spoons of Coffeemate instead (I like the taste)

Power-up spiced tea

A tea featuring a combination of spices, scientifically proven to aid in relieving fibromyalgia symptoms. This is my 'go-to' when my body is really run down or I get a bad cold.

Ingredients

Finger sized piece of ginger grated
2 tablespoons of fresh grated turmeric
1 piece of cinnamon bark
2 cloves
3 cups of water

Method

Bring all ingredients to boil for at least 15 minutes. Strain and serve.

Garlic tea

Most people find the idea of garlic revolting, and this creates a barrier in moving past the concept to a thing that can be helpful. I'll tell you what. This tea brought me great relief in the past when conventional medications took their time to work. I was very young (around 6 years old) when I started getting really sharp pains in the chest. I was diagnosed with Gastroesophageal reflux disease (GERD). For a digestive disorder this common, affecting 1 in 5 people in the UK, and over 60 million Americans, I've always felt like people don't understand the severity of the pain. I would be reeling in pain, folded in a ball in the wee hours of the morning for hours on end. My caring grandmother would find me and ask if I wanted to go to hospital. I was prescribed antacids but they took their time to work and the pain was too unbearable. In the following days I suffered from a sort of hang over effect, with a sore stomach, and unable to eat. I missed school, and in later years I was absent from work on account of this. What really helped and still helps me was my grandmother's garlic tea. In the beginning I was reluctant but she lovingly coaxed me into having a few sips, and in time I came to see garlic tea as a necessary 'evil'. The relief was much faster than the medications I took. It is imperative to note that as with many things in life, too much garlic can have the reverse effect on patients. Later in my twenties I was diagnosed with gastritis which I am also treated for. Garlic tea is an effective short term measure. In the long term, diet management is crucial to getting a hold on this condition. I ate strictly according to a list that my doctor provided, on the foods that I should avoid. This included peppermint, spicy foods (not an easy feat living in an East Indian household where spice ruled our meals), tomatoes, chocolate, citrus, and coffee. This is not an exhaustive list but more information can be found online on the NHS website or webmd.com. Sticking to this list has made me feel a lot better, and I'm now able to be more flexible with my diet while still managing it carefully.

Ingredients

3 cloves garlic
3 cups water

Method

Peel garlic and crush

Add to pot of water and bring to boil. Let it simmer for about 10 minutes.

Add a splash of milk (or cheat like me with a few spoons of Coffee mate) and a half spoon of sugar.

N.B. The milk and sugar are not necessary but my grandmother added them to improve the taste of the drink.

Caribbean style mackerel

Ingredients

5 medium mackerel, cleaned, rinsed and dried

For seasoning:
5 tablespoons of chopped coriander
1 tsp curry power
1 tsp geera
1 peg of garlic
1 tsp salt
1 tablespoon of lime juice
Optional: half of a scotch bonnet pepper

Method

Blend all seasoning ingredients. If you need more liquid to encourage the blending process, add a little vinegar

Make a few slashes diagonally along each fish and season with mixture thoroughly

On a baking dish, arrange enough foil paper to fold over

Lay seasoned fish in foil and cover, slightly sealing the edges

Grill for about 20 minutes in oven 180 degrees Celcius

Serve with salad or baked sweet potatoes

Grandmum's pak choi

Ingredients

3 stalks of pakchoi
3 large ripe tomatoes
1 tablespoon olive oil
1 small onion
A knob of ginger, peeled and grated
1tsp pepper sauce (optional)
Salt to taste
Optional: 1 tsp soy sauce

Method

Wash pak choi thoroughly and cut off ends

Lay leaves on top of eachother and cut into thin strips

Heat olive oil in pot

Chop tomatoes, onions and ginger and sauté in pot

When the tomatoes are cooked, mash them a bit with a wooden spoon to get the juices out.

Throw in the pakchoi and mix with ingredients in the pot

Add salt and pepper to taste

Cover pot on a low heat and cook for 10 minutes or until pak choi is cooked through.

Service on a bed of wholegrain basmati rice or as a side dish

Vegetarian quiche without crust

Ingredients

1 tablespoon olive oil

1 large leek

2 ripe tomatoes

1 small onion

1 tablespoon chopped coriander

A handful of spinach leaves

2 small bell peppers

A handful of grated cheddar cheese

100 grams cottage cheese

3 large eggs

1 cup of soy milk

Salt to taste

Method

Sauté vegetables in a pot with oil until cooked through. Add salt (pepper optional)

Crack eggs into a large bowl. Add cheddar cheese to eggs, followed by cottage cheese and milk. Mix together

Grease baking dish with butter

Lay out cooked vegetables in the greased dish evenly

Pour milk and egg mixture over the vegetables evenly

Bake in pre-heated oven at 180 degrees Celcius for 30 minutes

Pumpkin Talkerie

Talkerie refers to a form of curry or side dish that is made in some Caribbean islands with East Indian heritage. It usually involves cooking down a vegetable or fruit with seasonings and curry spices like masalas or ground cumin. Pumpkin talkerie has been one of my favourites since childhood, and it is rich in magnesium, as well as vitamins A, B5, C, and E.

Ingredients

½ lb pumpkin or a large squash (peeled and sliced thinly)
2-3 pegs garlic (chopped)
1 small onion (chopped)
2 tablespoons chopped coriander
2 tsps geera (ground cumin)
Salt to taste
3 tbsps oil
Pepper (hot) sauce to taste (optional)

Method

Heat oil on medium fire.

When the oil is hot, toss in the sliced pumpkin. Turn properly then cover on a low to medium heat. Some pumpkins spring water, that's alright, just leave it to dry down. If the pumpkin is too dry, you can add a few drops of water.

When pumpkin is halfway cooked, throw in chopped onion, garlic, coriander and geera, and place the lid on the pan again. Cover and simmer on a low heat for another 5-10 minutes.

Season with salt and pepper sauce (or piece of hot pepper if you have at home)

Use a potato masher to mash the pumpkin, until it turns into a sort of puree. Serve with parathas, dhalpuri rotis or naan bread.

Healthy Tuna burgers

Ingredients

2 cans of tuna fish
1 clove of garlic
1 tsp ground cumin
1 small onion
Knob of ginger peeled and chopped finely
Handful of coriander leaves chopped finely
1 egg
Salt to taste
Flour for dusting
Olive Oil for frying
Optional: hot peppers or pepper sauce

Method

Put all ingredients except flour, and olive oil in blender or food processor and give them a whizz. I didn't do this the last time, I just chopped everything finely and mixed them thoroughly by hand.

Wet your hands and shape a handful of the tuna mixture into balls, then flatten gently with palms. Make the burgers as big or small as you like.

Dust the burgers in some flour.

Heat oil and fry until burgers get brown, then carefully flip over onto the next side and fry.

Place in paper towels to soak up any excess oil.

An alternative to frying is grilling the burgers in an oven for 3 minutes on each side.

Peanut, banana punch

In Trinidad we frequently make what we call peanut punch. It's just a smoothie that you might already be familiar with, but I have added some extra bits to make it more invigorating! One of the ingredients is cinnamon. This spice is known to improve brain function (we need it with the fibro fog!), reduce inflammation, and fight bacteria with its antioxidant effects.

Ingredients

2 tablespoons of full fat peanut butter

1 banana

½ tsp nutmeg

1 tsp cinnamon

1tsp fresh grated turmeric

2 cups soy milk

Method

Blend all ingredients together with ice and serve immediately.

The banana can be replaced with mango.

Lentil Soup

This is a personal favourite of mine and I like to change up the ingredients from time to time. You can potentially use whatever vegetables you have in your fridge.

Ingredients

1 onion
Knob of ginger, peeled and chopped in fine pieces
Handful of chopped coriander
½ tsp ground cumin
1 tsp turmeric
85 g brown lentils, rinsed
3 carrots sliced
1 stick celery or 1 large sweet potato
2 cups coconut milk
2 tablespoons olive oil
Salt to taste
Optional: hot pepper

Method

Heat the oil in a pot and add the onion, and ginger.

Saute the onion and ginger until the fragrances start coming out

Add the carrot and celery (or sweet potato, whichever you choose) and stir the pot.

Add the lentils, turmeric and coconut milk and cook until lentils are very soft and vegetables cooked through. Add a little water if required.

Add salt and ground cumin, and cook for another 5 minutes

Optional: You can whizz the soup with a hand blender or have as it is. This hearty soup is ideal for those down days when you need a boost or you're just feeling unwell.

Medication and Supplements

"It is part of the cure to wish to be cured" – Seneca

Since my diagnosis in 2010, I have been prescribed a variety of medications and supplements for fibromyalgia. The US Food and Drug Administration has only approved three drugs for the specific treatment of fibromyalgia. These are Pregabalin (Lyrica), Duloxetine (Cymbalta) and Milnacipran (Savella). These medications help to reduce pain in some people with fibromyalgia.

The very first medications I was started on were Amitriptyline, Citalopram, and Cocodamol. I found Amitryptaline quite good, particularly helping me to sleep at night. The other two did nothing for me really, except that Cocodamol made me nauseous. Later on, I moved onto Tramadol, Duloxetine and Pregabalin, the latter I still take with Propranolol, Omeprazole for my gastritis and acid reflux, and Mirtazapine for depression (useful in helping me sleep!).

Over the years in support groups and my own family circles, I have been challenged on taking medications for fibromyalgia. The question has always been whether we can justify taking the medications that we do. Often, people cite the side effects or speculate that the medications aren't helping anyway so why bother.

Before I started medication for fibromyalgia I struggled with coping every day. Some days I couldn't lift myself up from bed, and I experienced more frequent episodes of sleep paralysis or what I refer to as my body shutting down in the most inappropriate of times. Studying and working were ten times harder. I have suffered from some side effects like an increase in my weight, but I have gained more than I've lost. When I consider how fibromyalgia steals our dreams and lives, I staunchly decided that I would rather have some quality of life on medication than have a longer life in a worse off position. I understand that some patients cope without medications but in all the support groups I have come across, I found these patients to be in the minority. It is tough tackling the myriad of symptoms that fibromyalgia throws our way, and most of us need whatever help we can get.

With medication and lifestyle changes I manage to have some quality of life with functionality, compared to my bedridden past. I suppose this is a very personal issue that each of us has to answer ourselves. Each of us has to do what is best for us because we are the ones enduring this nightmare every day.

I also take a number of supplements recommended by doctors and other patients. These include:

- Peppermint capsules for IBS
- Fennel seed capsules to reduce bloating associated with IBS
- Acidophilus capsules to promote healthy bacteria in the gut for IBS symptoms
- Magnesium supplements for pain and fatigue
- Multivitamins
- Vitamins B Complex, E, C, D, zinc, cranberry, selenium and magnesium supplements
- Co-enzyme Q10 for fatigue, antioxidant, immune, and muscular support.
- Glucosamine supplements for keeping joint cartilage healthy
- Omega 3 fish oil capsules for healthy muscles and mood
- D-ribose for energy levels

Lifestyle

"It's never too late, it's never too bad and you're never too old or too sick to start from scratch once again" – Bikram Choudhury

I think this will likely be one of the hardest bits to consider in aiming for a better life, and possibly the best life with fibromyalgia. They say it takes sixty-six days for new behaviour to become automatic, or in other words, for us to form a new habit. I often start off all hot and sweaty, lose momentum and then before I can say 'she sells sea shells on the sea shore', I'm back into my old ways. Remember if it's worth fighting for (and your health and life are definitely worth it!) then it will likely require great effort. It isn't easy but we can do it.

Get your diet in order

As previously mentioned I have started trying out the ketogenic diet. This is an important part of my lifestyle. I often slip up but at least I try to restrict my diet to natural, unprocessed foods. You don't have to adopt this diet but you will need to take a proper inspection of your eating habits. I would encourage you to try to eat fresh, healthy and natural foods. If you can't cook, now is a great time to start learning too. The BBC recipes website is a useful resource for cooking all kinds of foods[7]. At least, you'll know what's in your food.

Don't comfort eat

I know first-hand that living with a chronic illness can sometimes encourage us into comfort eating; it is something I struggle with terribly. But the more I comfort eat, the more weight I gain and the harder it is to move around freely. My knees and legs become weaker and I am more inclined to stay in bed. Not good at all. So it is imperative that we put a lid on that, and make sure that we are in charge, so the food is not controlling us!

Epsom salts baths

This is another old family remedy that has been around for as long as I can remember. When I forgot, my paternal grandmother was there to remind me. Ideally this should be done as often as possible. Baths usually make me feel much more exhausted so I don't do it as often as possible but when I do I never, ever regret it. My grandmother tells me to run the water as hot as I can take it (this usually depends on my pain levels) and pour a generous amount of Epsom salts in

---

7   bbc.co.uk/food/recipes

the water. I usually use about a heaped handful of the salts, and I pour it in just before I step into the water. I soak in the tub for at least 30 minutes, and I find this particularly helpful when my muscles are sore and achy. It also helps me with getting some sleep, a rarity for us fibromyalgia patients. Epsom salts are packed with magnesium, which is highly rated for promoting the proper function of muscles and nerves among other things.

Get out and about (exercise is a must)

After I graduated, I was looking for a job for quite a while, and found myself becoming one with my bed. It became harder and harder to get out in the mornings, which are most difficult for me. I totally understand the struggle that accompanies pain and debilitating exhaustion. I needed something to get me out of bed, because I was getting entangled in a vicious cycle that perpetuated itself. I started gaining a lot of weight and at the time it was already excruciatingly painful to walk. On a good day I could barely manage five steps without limping. I was often in tears as a result. The soles of my feet were constantly sore and painful, and my GP was saying something about steroid injections, followed by possible surgery on my feet. I was terrified to say the least. I'll take needles anywhere, but not under my feet matey. I was shaken into action. It was suggested that I get a walking stick. I was 26 going on 96.

I had read over and over again about how exercise was compulsory in the treatment of fibromyalgia, but I couldn't understand how this would work when any exercise left me with a flare of pain and bed ridden in the following days. Most other fms patients I knew reported the same. I think an emphasis needs to be placed on graded exercise for fibromyalgia patients. That is, structured exercise programmes to meet the needs of the patient.

I started physiotherapy once a week but the hard bit was being motivated enough to do the exercises on my own at home. I would stand on the edge of the stairs in my house, holding the banister, tiptoeing up and down slowly. Before I could reach twenty I would call it quits. I cannot tell you how frustrated I was. I know you know. My physiotherapist made it clear that I had to do the work for me. It was going to hurt but I needed to do it.

I realise that period was like most things in life. Sometimes it gets worse before it gets better. Along with my frequent Epsom salts baths, I continued physiotherapy and changed my diet to healthy, fresh foods.

Then something else happened. I got a job. That job forced me out of bed every single day. I needed work to pay the bills but I dreaded it. My neighbourhood birds who I secretly fed would be beckoning in the morning, and I would be cursing my alarm clock. Little sleep, severe exhaustion and pain were there with me every single morning, but that job got me out of bed. I rolled myself out of bed, crawled when I had to. That was the most important part, because if I didn't get out of that bed, the longer I stayed, the harder it became to get up, and I was more likely to call in sick. That job forced me to get some of the only exercise I was getting. Rushing for the bus or train, and walking around the office might sound like nothing but it was definitely something. I really really believe it was that combination of physiotherapy, Epsom salt baths, healthy eating, and that job that got my feet better. I never subjected myself to those steroid injections under my feet and hell no to that surgery as well. My feet are so much better now that I cannot overstate the value in finding something to get you out of bed and about daily.

Maybe you can't work but you can consider doing a part time voluntary role. It should be something that you will feel a sense of obligation to. Every single day when I have to get out of bed it is hard. It is the same struggle. Sometimes I oversleep, sometimes I don't hear my four alarms or my friend phoning to wake me, and some days I cannot get up, yes. I'm not very motivated to do it because of the level of pain and exhaustion I am in, but I have to do it and ultimately it has been good for me. Sometimes it is hard to do the things that are good for us, but like a caring parent who knows what's best for their child, we have to be that to ourselves. People sometimes tell me I shouldn't be working and

I really do push myself to the limit just to cope, but I tell you, working is one of the best management methods I've used in tackling the fibro monster. Getting out and about is a must! Additionally, I realise it helps add structure to my day. When I am not working, anything goes and that lack of structure creates more problems than anything else.

Nap

Napping has become an important coping mechanism for me. I think it is imperative to listen to our bodies. I can't do it in the middle of the day if I'm at work but if my body is saying it really needs a rest, as soon as I get home I plan for it. I try to have dinner and then a nap or if I have to I just head straight for the bed and then have dinner later on.

When I am in more pain than usual, it becomes easier for me to stay in bed all day. The temptation is ever present but personally I feel it does more harm than good. If I stay in bed all day my muscles and joints get weaker, I particularly feel it in my knees. Then when I have to walk I find that my legs and feet are reluctant to listen to my instructions. They feel heavy. It is always difficult and scary for me when that happens because it reminds me of where I was years ago when the simple activity of walking was so distressing. I definitely do not want to go back there. So as tough as it is, even when I am experiencing an exacerbation of symptoms,

I try not to stay in bed all day. A little stretch every couple hours, a walk, or a soak in the tub with Epsom salts all help.

Pace yourself

It would be remiss of me not to mention the importance of pacing yourself in any activity you pursue. You have to know how much you can manage, and not overwork yourself. It's a problem many of us have. When we have our bad days and we're bed bound, we often worry about all the work that's piling up. So when our good days come, we think that we need to get as much done possible. The danger in this is that we risk overworking ourselves, and we're likely to end up suffering a flare of symptoms in the following days. The Macmillan Dictionary says to 'pace yourself' is "to avoid doing something too quickly or doing too much at one time so that you have enough energy left to complete an activity." Due to our low levels of energy and limiting symptoms which affect our ability to function daily, pacing ourselves is a vital part of our lives.

Managing stress

Like pacing ourselves, managing our stress levels is equally significant in the management of fibromyalgia. Many of us experience an exacerbation of our symptoms, often becoming anxious when we get stressed over events in our lives.

This is an area of my life that I am constantly working on, because I suffer heightened anxiety levels, migraines, pain, depression, dizziness and cognitive impairments when I am too stressed. It's impossible to avoid stress entirely but if we can, we should try to remove ourselves from stressful situations, or people who make us feel that way. If we can't, when stressful situations arise, we should try to manage our emotions, and see the events as inconvenient but manageable situations, which will work out in the end. Of course sometimes we have to take action to ensure things do work out ultimately, the crucial bit is trying to stay calm the whole while. It's helpful if you have an understanding friend who will support you throughout. It's tough I know, especially in the case of longstanding problems but it's possible, and you'll learn more about the tools I use for this, in the next chapter.

Bikram yoga

I never thought I would have done it, but I had started going out with Paul, who was a strong advocate of Bikram Yoga. I find it hard to stay still and yoga never really appealed to me. The truth is I never really believed that it could help me. Paul persuaded me to try it out and the next thing I know I was sitting in a classroom of 40 degrees Celsius with other yogis going through twenty-six postures. Each class lasts 90 minutes and more than often I couldn't do every posture. It was exhausting but I cannot lie, from the very first day I did it, I noticed certain benefits. My irritable bowel syndrome symptoms had improved drastically! My symptoms of bloating and constipation had eased significantly. I was able to get better sleep in the night, which was a big deal considering that I've suffered from terrible insomnia since childhood. It also helped me to manage a healthy weight with the little exercise I got, and with taking medication with weight gain side effects. Those were the direct benefits that I experienced, but Bikram Yoga is touted for lots of other advantages including detoxification, which happens as a result of the heavy sweating.

Look, I can imagine how intimidating the idea must be, I totally understand. I didn't think I could do it and it was challenging yes. The point is I did do it, I tried as best as I possibly could and that is all we can do. I never thought I would manage with the temperature as I suffered terribly when I lived in Trinidad with its daily 32 degrees Celcius. I often passed out and dizziness plagued me. I had moments of that in Bikram yoga but the class receives great advice on how to manage any challenges. With a higher intake of water and eating properly, I ensured that I gave myself the best shot of managing the classes. It's definitely worth a try.

Acupuncture

I won't talk about this much because I'm still traumatised. I had roughly six sessions which had started off fairly alright. I didn't see any improvements but it was suggested that I needed to do a course of it before seeing the true benefits. The last sessions were horrific and the needles in my knees hurt so badly I cried. When they came out and the therapist massaged me, I repeatedly asked him to be gentler as my body was so sore and painful but both my cries and pleas were in vain. Needless to say, that was the last time I did acupuncture.

Wong to Yick Woodlock Medicated Balm Oil

Back when I was doing my Masters Degree my pain levels were so high and I suffered most with my legs and feet. I was in a really dark place. All my university mates were going to classes and managing active social lives in the magical city that is London. But I was never there with them. I was so knackered all the time but more than that walking was just too darn painful. Then I stumbled across this herbal Chinese oil in a shop close to where I was living. It was a risk buying it at £9.00 but I have never regretted it. This worked wonders in tandem with other things like my Epsom salt baths. I even bought it for both my grandmothers who live with severe arthritis and they both reported an improvement in their pain levels. You can find it in many Chinese supermarkets and from online retailers like Amazon.

When I'm out of Woodlock Oil I run to Phorpain gel which, unlike other muscle rubs, doesn't burn my skin and actually helps alleviate the pain.

Cognitive Behavioural Therapy (CBT)

Cognitive Behavioural Therapy can be useful in the treatment of some conditions including depression and anxiety, which many fibromyalgia patients live with. I did it for seven months but ultimately the therapist and I agreed that it was not the most suitable therapy for me. It did however help me to understand more about the way that I think, and how to effectively manage my problems by challenging ways of thinking. If you also struggle with managing stress in your life, CBT may be useful in helping you to manage it.

Psychotherapy

Aside from the fact that depression and anxiety are common symptoms among many of us, a lot of fibromyalgia patients I talk to deal with difficult relationships and painful emotions. Psychotherapy can be very useful in providing an outlet for us to not only vent but learn skills and techniques to manage difficult relationships and our own emotions. It is hard work but beneficial in many ways. I know.

Other helpful tools and tips

Insoles

Remember those years of painful walking? Well what also helped me through was wearing insoles in my shoes. The physiotherapist had found that apart from fibromyalgia, I was also living with plantar fasctis and a mid tarsal sprain, which caused a severe burning pain under my feet every morning, or when I lay down. She had suggested that I get special orthotics made but in the interim advised that I could get a pair over the counter. I paid around £25.00 for a pair of Scholl Orthaheel Heel and Ankle Stabiliser from Boots pharmacy. At first they felt a bit uncomfortable but they greatly eased the pressure and severe discomfort in my feet. What's also important is that they've lasted quite long, considering that I used them every single day.

Meaningful Living

"Only a life lived for others is worth living" – *Albert Einstein*

"I have found that among its other benefits, giving liberates the soul of the giver" – *Maya Angelo*

One of the most powerful things in life is to witness someone in the throes of darkness, putting their heart towards making life better for another human being.

There is power in living life for others; to make it better for them, even when we need help ourselves.

I never really thought I had anything to give. I mean, I could barely take care of myself, and required the support of others to cope. What difference could I possibly make to anyone else? I suppose when I thought of giving, I automatically thought of handing money to a homeless person or financially contributing in some way. I have however learnt that giving goes far beyond money and material things. I learned to give my time, my ears, empathy, and I learned the power of sharing my story to encourage others. That was what made a difference to me in my time of need, and I decided that I would do it for others too. The reason I'm telling you this is because giving to others has given me reason to plod on even in the deepest pits of life. I can't really explain the science behind how it works but I know that it works.

You see, I had come from a place where there was little empathy. I reached out for help for depression, post traumatic stress disorder and fibromyalgia, but often the response was dismissive. At times my outpouring was met by silence or complete disregard of what I had said. This was what I got from the people in my life. It was heartbreaking, and it hardened my heart against humanity. I had been shown more love by my pet parrots!

In 2013, depression was winning its war against me. The thin threads I was hanging from were on the brink of breaking and I was ready to give in. I was fed up of being empty and hollow on the inside, tired of fibromyalgia stealing my dreams and walking this long road alone. It was one of the worse years of my life, but also one of the most important. I learnt a number of life changing lessons. Anyone could have told me and I might have read some of it in self-help books, but the lessons wouldn't have had the impact unless I had experienced them myself. I am not an advocate of suicide but I am not one of those persons who hands down judgement to our friends, who have ended their lives. I know what it is like to be in such unbearable pain, pain that breaks you and sucks the life from you; Pain that binds you so badly that you become desperate for an escape. You hold on until you can't any longer. And for those of our friends who gave up, it was because this life became too agonizing, and death seemingly offered a door to a place where there would be no pain. That is the extent of desperation experienced. Many fibromyalgia patients I know have gone through this. I too have been there, and I still fight it every single day.

That year, a lot of my support came from Depression Alliance (DA), a charity that supports people living with depression. I am a member of DA, who I also volunteer with. I host activities to raise money for this charity, and I also help to raise awareness of depression. I have a blog that focuses on living with fibromyalgia and depression. It has made all the difference in my battle with these two conditions. During the depressive episodes of 2013, I had locked myself away from the world, but friends from DA responded with exceptional kindness, sending help my way and never judging me. It was too much for my mind to fathom.

"The giving of love is an education in itself" – Eleanor Roosevelt

Following my discharge from hospital, I was unable to venture out to collect my medication. A fellow DA member who I had never met in person, collected my medication and brought them home to me. She came with her sister, and they stayed and encouraged me. It was hard to understand how someone I had never met could show me such love and kindness. Other friends from the charity who I had known only through email exchanges and forum chats, phoned my GP, followed up on me daily, and did just about anything to provide the practical support that I needed. This outpouring of love helped me in so many ways, because I saw that while I was too weak to fight for myself other people were willing to fight for me. When I got better, I decided to do the same for others. I noticed the change in me.

Numerous studies[8] have indicated that charitable giving is beneficial to our health, decreasing pain in patients with chronic illnesses due to the release of endorphins. Giving to others not only makes us happy but alleviates stress and connects us with people in an amazing way.[9] I absolutely love this because I can testify to it!

Helping others encouraged me to plod on because it also took the focus away from my own pain. I felt motivated to go to the aid of others because I have lived through life changing pain, and I don't want anyone else to experience this.

---

8   oprah.com/health/Scientific-Proof-That-Charitable-Giving-Improves-Your-Health_1

9   greatergood.berkeley.edu/article/item/5_ways_giving_is_good_for_you

Hope & resolve not to give up

"Out of suffering have emerged the strongest souls; the most massive characters are seared with scars" – Khalil Gibran

We all have our moments when we feel like throwing in the towel. This is one of my biggest challenges, also faced by many fibromyalgia patients. Depression is a common symptom of fibromyalgia. No surprise there, it's not easy living in pain or trying to live in the wreckage of our lives. Many of our fibromyalgia friends live without support as well.

In some of my most despairing moments, some of the strongest advice I've received has come from my paternal grandmother, who has persevered through a life of hardships. Mama Claire's message is always consistent.

"I am older so I've endured more. So I know. I know that things will work out in the end but for that to happen you cannot give up" she said to me in 2013. "I am going down but I'm still fighting."

Of course it's easier said than done but we can do it by taking it one small step at a time. It's helpful to talk to someone with perspective. I mean someone like my Mama Claire who has been there, and lived to tell the tale. Without hope there is nothing to live for. Hope is what gets us out of bed in the mornings, what pushes us to carry on when we are down to our very last. Even if we don't recognise it, most of us live with some degree of hope. Hope is what keeps us, and it is important to nurture that seed.

I have accepted that it will be very difficult for me to pursue my dreams of traditional journalism due to the cognitive and physical challenges associated with fibromyalgia, but there is no way I am giving up on all my dreams. You shouldn't either. I sat myself down, and tried to think of how I could practise journalism, while making accommodations for my health. There is more than one way of doing something. No matter how bad it is, there is always something that we can still do. We human beings have so much to give. The thing about this life is we have only one shot. Life won't ease up on us because we have fibromyalgia, so we have to give it our best with what we have. Even if it takes us twice as long, with ten times more fight, we should never give up on our dreams. Crowded House's *Don't Dream It's Over*, made popular by Sixpence None the Richer, has always resonated with me for that reason.

Empathy

"Empathy is a choice and it is vulnerable choice because in order to connect with you, I have to connect with something in myself that knows that feeling" – Dr Brene Brown.

Connecting and empathising with other fibromyalgia patients or those one can relate to not only support the other person, but they remind us that we are not alone in our journey. Empathy is an important part of our humanity. Professor Brown explains the power of empathy in an amazing video available on her website.[10] Find it on Youtube by searching for Brene Brown on Empathy.

Have faith

"Faith consists of believing when it is beyond the power of reason to believe" – Voltaire

Living in faith can make all the difference in our struggles with health. My grandmother is a praying woman, and always says to me "when you're just about to go under, He will reach out in the nick of time, and lift you up." I always say on my blog that this is not a lesson in religion. Faith is knowing that things will be alright despite what lays before us; it is believing in our hearts that we will overcome even though we cannot see how. For this to work however we can't just sit back and wait. We have to work. We have to act on our belief. We cannot get back something from giving nothing. I will say it again, life doesn't give us a break because we suffer.

---

10 theinvisiblef.com/2014/01/13/being-empathetic

I wanted to publish my first novel but I couldn't see how I was going to do it. Completing the story was a big challenge. In the three years of working on it on and off, I had had two major nervous breakdowns and serious difficulties with my health. When I finally finished I had been rejected time after time by all the big name publishers. I felt dejected. I really wanted it to happen so I decided to make it happen. I learnt about self publishing, and it took me a while to digest everything because of the cognitive challenges we face with fibromyalgia. It took me a lot longer than it does most authors but in the end I achieved my goal!

Have faith, believe and work without ceasing. We are not our disability. Fibromyalgia doesn't define us. We define ourselves. I understand it is a bold statement to make in light of how debilitating and encompassing this condition is. The trouble is, the moment we let fms define us, we throw our lives at its mercy. Anything is possible if we believe and work hard. Say to yourself 'I am not fibromyalgia and fibromyalgia is not me!' One day when a cure is found for fibromyalgia we don't want to look back and think 'if only I hadn't given up, I would have been at this place or at this position in my life.' Take your time with whatever it is you want to pursue. Take your whole life to do it if you must, the point is to keep pushing ahead. Use this challenge as a stepping stone. Think of our obstacles as stones, piling up one on the other. We just have to keep on climbing up that mountain of stones. Never stop climbing. When you succeed, your victory will be all the sweeter because you, only you will know how much you gave and sacrificed. Sometimes our biggest challenges can be our biggest motivators. We never know what is around the corner because we cannot see the end from the beginning. It's hard but that's where faith comes in.

Laugh

I got caught up in my suffering; in the daily pain and struggles with fibro fog, fatigue, dizziness and the whole lot of it. I forgot to smile. Sometimes we don't always notice when pain starts changing us. We can become irritable and unhappy all the time. It's a cycle, and the more we become negative that feeds into itself. It really helps to try and laugh at the little things. To notice the beauty around us and smile even when it is hard. On my blog I talk about pretending myself better. It is really me making a concerted effort to smile and feel better even though I feel like a crumbling tower. The cycle works in the reverse too. The more I smile and laugh, the more positivity I seem to attract. Ever so often I will still have to deal with negative people, but that affects me less once the positivity chain starts kicking in. Try it. When you feel like crying or getting angry, just smile.

Take your focus away from the thing hurting you, and find something light and beautiful to look at.

Avoid the doubters and negativity

This isn't always the easiest thing to do, especially when we are talking about family or people close to us. Perhaps my most painful experience with this was someone in my life who severely criticised me, and even made fun of how exhausted and dizzy I was all the time. Over the years I have had to weed out the negative people from my life, one by one. You know, the people who don't believe that you're in pain or the ones judging you because you don't live a typical life. I have heard so many stories from fms patients who have been accused of faking their symptoms, the accusations coming from loved ones and medical professionals. Firstly, I try to give people a chance. I explain and point them to legitimate sources of information on fibromyalgia. If they remain sceptical and judgemental, then move on. If it's a medical practitioner telling me it's all in my head, then I don't see them again. I feel much lighter without all that negativity in my life and so will you. I really feel this is key to living the best life with fms. We need to do as much as we can to avoid and alleviate stress in our lives, as this causes a flare in our symptoms. Surround yourself with people who empathise and show you kindness. I have some friends who may not entirely understand how fibromyalgia affects me but the crucial thing is that they don't judge me, they listen and show me support.

Summary

We can become comfortable with our pain. We get so used to living in pain, day in day out that we do more than just accept it in our lives. We start letting it rule our lives – what we do, where we go, which of our dreams we pursue, and which we pack away. In a sense, I can understand why we do this. But fibromyalgia doesn't have to control our lives. We need to step out of that complacency and take our lives back.

Regaining control over our lives can start in many ways, some of which I've outlined in this book. They include reviewing our diets to ensure we're eating healthily, and consuming foods that will fight against fibromyalgia. I also discussed the importance of connecting with others, giving, avoiding negative people, finding something to get us out of bed daily, and overall meaningful living.

There is no one size-fits-all solution to fibromyalgia. It affects every patient differently, and what works for one might not work for another. The solutions in this book are what worked for me. They may or may not work for you but you never know unless you try. Again, please remember I am not a medical practitioner. The advice given in this work is based on my personal experiences, and old natural remedies handed down by my grandparents.

I end by encouraging you to hope and live for love. Of all the remedies mentioned, I place emphasis on these. We need hope to keep pushing us forward, to remind us that even though we cannot see through the darkness, there is light ahead. On love, what else can I say? It is the ultimate source of power. After we have been touched by love, we can never be the same. It's important that we not only receive it, but that we willingly give it too. If you listen to nothing else I've said, please heed these last words. Love always finds a way. This is the end product of living for others. There you will find an infinite source of the power that you need.

"The purpose of life is not to be happy. It is to be useful, to be honourable, to be compassionate, to have it make some difference that you have lived and lived well"
– Ralph Waldo Emerson

Acknowledgements

To my blog followers whose constant, positive feedback encouraged me to pen this little handbook.

I'm thankful to my dear friend Susan Jacobs for her unfailing kindness and support, and for showing me great empathy even when she is battling the fibromyalgia monster.

To those doctors and researchers who spend their time and efforts working on our behalf to make things better for us, in the hope that one day we will find a cure.

Lastly, but certainly not least, to my Lord for His goodness and favour.

Gentle hugs :)

About the Author

Alisha Nurse grew up on the Caribbean island of Trinidad. She holds an MA in International Journalism from the University of Westminster, London.

She loves curry, sharing stories and talking to random people on public transportation.

Alisha lives with fibromyalgia and clinical depression, and is keen to raise awareness. She blogs about her experiences at theinvisiblef.com.

Her debut novel, an early teen fantasy story *The Return of the Key* is available from Amazon.com and other online retailers. Her website is authoralishanurse.com.

Printed in Great Britain
by Amazon

68738945R00047